Body Weight Exercise Made Easy Guide for Beginners

Understanding the Essential of Body Weight Exercises

By

Smiddy Tiberius

Table of Contents

CHAPTER 1

Introduction

1.1 Why Body Weight Exercises?

Body weight exercises are a fundamental component of any fitness regimen, and they offer a compelling and accessible way for individuals to improve their strength, flexibility, and overall physical health. The appeal of body weight exercises lies in their simplicity and convenience, making them an excellent choice for beginners and experienced fitness enthusiasts alike.

One of the primary reasons why body weight exercises are so popular is that they require minimal equipment or none at all. You don't need a gym membership or expensive weights to get started. All you need is your own body and a bit of space to move. This accessibility means that body weight exercises can be performed virtually anywhere, whether you're at home, in a park, or while traveling. As a result, they break down barriers to entry into the world of fitness and make it easy for individuals to engage in physical activity on their own terms.

Additionally, body weight exercises are incredibly versatile and can be adapted to suit various fitness levels and goals. Whether you're looking to build strength, increase endurance, enhance flexibility, or lose weight, there are body weight exercises suitable for your needs. Beginners can start with basic movements and gradually progress to more challenging ones as they gain confidence and strength. On the other hand, seasoned athletes can use advanced variations of body weight exercises to maintain and fine-tune their fitness.

Beyond their accessibility and adaptability, body weight exercises offer a holistic approach to fitness. They engage multiple muscle groups simultaneously, helping to improve overall functional strength and balance. Unlike some isolated weightlifting exercises that focus on specific muscle groups, body weight exercises promote a more balanced and integrated development of the body. This not only leads to better physical performance but also reduces the risk of imbalances and injuries.

1.2 Benefits of Body Weight Exercises

The benefits of incorporating body weight exercises into your fitness routine are multifaceted and extend far beyond just physical fitness. These exercises offer a host of advantages that can positively impact various aspects of your life:

1. **Cost-Effective:** As mentioned earlier, body weight exercises require little to no equipment. This makes them an affordable option for anyone, eliminating the need for costly gym memberships or expensive exercise machines.

2. **Convenience:** You can perform body weight exercises anywhere, anytime. Whether you're at home, in a hotel room, or at a local park, you can maintain your fitness routine with ease.

3. **Improved Strength:** Body weight exercises challenge your muscles in a functional and balanced way, enhancing overall strength. These exercises help develop not only individual muscle groups but also the

coordination and synergy between them.

4. **Enhanced Flexibility:** Many body weight exercises involve stretching and dynamic movements, promoting increased flexibility and joint mobility.

5. **Weight Management:** Regular engagement in body weight exercises can help with weight management and fat loss, as they increase your metabolic rate and improve muscle mass.

6. **Cardiovascular Health:** Certain body weight exercises, like burpees or jumping jacks, can serve as effective cardio workouts, benefiting heart health and endurance.

7. **No Special Skills Required:** Unlike some sports or activities that may require specialized skills

or equipment, body weight exercises are accessible to individuals of all fitness levels and abilities.

8. **Injury Prevention:** Body weight exercises can contribute to injury prevention by strengthening muscles and improving stability and flexibility, reducing the risk of common injuries.

9. **Enhanced Body Awareness:** These exercises encourage better mind-muscle connection, helping you become more aware of your body and how it moves.

10. **Stress Reduction:** Engaging in physical activity, even if it's just a short body weight workout, can help reduce stress and improve mental well-being.

11. **Long-Term Sustainability:** Since body weight exercises are

low-impact and adaptable, they can be part of a sustainable, lifelong fitness regimen that evolves with your changing needs and goals.

body weight exercises are a versatile and accessible way to improve your physical health and overall well-being. Whether you're a beginner looking to start your fitness journey or an experienced athlete seeking a well-rounded workout routine, body weight exercises offer numerous benefits that can enhance your quality of life. Their simplicity, convenience, and adaptability make them an excellent choice for individuals of all backgrounds and fitness levels.

CHAPTER 2

Getting Started

2.1 Setting Clear Goals

Before embarking on a body weight exercise routine, it's essential to set clear and achievable goals. Having well-defined objectives can provide you with motivation, direction, and a sense of purpose in your fitness journey. Here are some tips on how to set clear goals:

1. **Specificity:** Your goals should be specific rather than vague. For example, instead of saying, "I want to get fit," specify, "I want to be able to do 20 push-ups without resting."

2. **Measurable:** Make your goals measurable, so you can track your

progress. This could involve counting repetitions, measuring time, or monitoring improvements in flexibility or body composition.

3. **Achievable:** Ensure that your goals are realistic and attainable based on your current fitness level. Setting overly ambitious goals can lead to frustration or even injury.

4. **Relevant:** Your goals should align with your personal values and desires. Consider why you want to achieve a particular goal and how it will positively impact your life.

5. **Time-Bound:** Set a timeframe for achieving your goals. For example, "I want to achieve 10 consecutive pull-ups within three months."

6. **Write Them Down:** Putting your goals in writing can make them feel more concrete and increase your commitment to achieving them.

7. **Short-Term and Long-Term Goals:** Include both short-term goals (weeks to a few months) and long-term goals (months to years) in your plan. Short-term goals act as stepping stones toward your ultimate objectives.

2.2 Safety Precautions

Safety is of paramount importance when engaging in any exercise routine, including body weight exercises. Here are some safety precautions to keep in mind:

1. **Consult with a Healthcare Professional:** If you have any underlying medical conditions,

are new to exercise, or have concerns about your health, it's advisable to consult with a healthcare professional or physician before starting a new workout program.

2. **Proper Form:** Pay close attention to your form when performing body weight exercises. Incorrect form can lead to injuries. It's often helpful to learn the proper technique from a qualified trainer or reliable online resources.

3. **Start Slowly:** If you're a beginner, start with easier variations of exercises and gradually progress to more challenging ones. Overexerting yourself in the beginning can lead to muscle soreness and potential injuries.

4. **Listen to Your Body:** Be attuned to your body's signals. If you

experience pain, discomfort, or dizziness during an exercise, stop immediately and assess the situation. Don't push through severe pain.

5. **Warm-Up:** Always begin your workout with a proper warm-up to prepare your muscles and joints for exercise. A warm-up can consist of light cardiovascular activities like jogging in place or jumping jacks, along with dynamic stretching.

6. **Cool-Down:** After your workout, engage in a cool-down routine that includes static stretching to help your muscles recover and reduce the risk of post-exercise soreness.

7. **Hydration:** Stay hydrated throughout your workout to prevent dehydration. Dehydration

can affect your performance and overall well-being.

8. **Rest:** Your body needs time to recover, so avoid overtraining. Adequate rest between workout sessions is crucial for muscle recovery and growth.

9. **Footwear and Clothing:** Wear appropriate workout attire and comfortable footwear to prevent slips, blisters, or other discomfort during exercise.

2.3 Basic Warm-Up and Cool-Down

Warming up and cooling down are essential components of any exercise routine, and body weight exercises are no exception. Here's a basic warm-up and cool-down routine to incorporate into your workouts:

Warm-Up:

1. **Jumping Jacks:** 2-3 minutes of jumping jacks to elevate your heart rate and warm up your entire body.

2. **Arm Circles:** Stand with your arms extended to the sides and make circular motions with your arms for 30 seconds in each direction.

3. **Leg Swings:** Hold onto a stable support and swing one leg forward and backward, then side to side, for about 30 seconds per leg.

4. **Torso Twists:** Stand with your feet hip-width apart and twist your torso from side to side for 30 seconds.

5. **Dynamic Stretching:** Perform dynamic stretches such as leg swings, hip circles, and arm

swings for 3-5 minutes to gradually increase joint mobility and flexibility.

Cool-Down:

1. **Static Stretches:** Stretch the major muscle groups you've worked during your workout. Hold each stretch for 15-30 seconds without bouncing.

2. **Deep Breathing:** Take a few minutes to focus on deep, diaphragmatic breathing to help your body relax and recover.

3. **Hydration:** Rehydrate with water to replace fluids lost during exercise.

Incorporating these warm-up and cool-down routines into your body weight exercise regimen will help reduce the risk of injury, improve flexibility, and enhance overall workout effectiveness. Remember, safety and injury prevention

are key priorities as you begin your
fitness journey.

CHAPTER 3

Essential Body Weight Exercises

3.1 Push-Ups

Push-ups are a classic and highly effective body weight exercise that primarily target the chest, shoulders, and triceps, while also engaging the core and back muscles. They are an essential exercise for building upper body strength and can be modified to suit different fitness levels.

How to Perform Push-Ups:

1. Begin in a plank position with your hands placed slightly wider than shoulder-width apart.

2. Keep your body in a straight line from head to heels, engaging your core for stability.

3. Lower your chest toward the ground by bending your elbows. Your elbows should be at around a 45-degree angle to your body.

4. Keep your body in a straight line as you lower and then push back up to the starting position, fully extending your arms.

Variations:

- **Incline Push-Ups:** Place your hands on an elevated surface, like a bench or a sturdy table, to make the exercise easier.

- **Knee Push-Ups:** Perform push-ups with your knees on the ground, which reduces the resistance and is suitable for beginners.

- **Diamond Push-Ups:** Place your hands close together under your chest to emphasize triceps engagement.

3.2 Squats

Squats are a fundamental lower body exercise that target the quadriceps, hamstrings, glutes, and lower back. They are excellent for building leg strength and enhancing overall lower body function.

How to Perform Squats:

1. Stand with your feet shoulder-width apart, toes pointing slightly outward.

2. Keep your chest up and your back straight as you lower your body by bending your knees and hips.

3. Lower yourself until your thighs are parallel to the ground or as far as your mobility allows.

4. Push through your heels to return to the starting position.

Variations:

- **Body Weight Squats:** The basic squat without any added resistance.

- **Goblet Squats:** Hold a weight (e.g., a dumbbell or kettlebell) close to your chest while squatting.

- **Pistol Squats:** An advanced variation where you perform squats on one leg, extending the other leg forward.

3.3 Planks

Planks are an exceptional body weight exercise for strengthening the core, including the abdominal muscles, obliques, lower back, and stabilizing muscles. They help improve posture and provide a strong foundation for many other exercises.

How to Perform Planks:

1. Start in a push-up position with your forearms on the ground, elbows directly beneath your shoulders.

2. Keep your body in a straight line from head to heels, engaging your core and glutes.

3. Hold this position for as long as you can, maintaining proper form. Avoid sagging or raising your hips.

Variations:

- **Side Planks:** Rotate your body to one side, balancing on one forearm, and engage your oblique muscles.

- **Plank Leg Lifts:** Lift one leg off the ground while in the plank position, alternating between legs.

- **Plank With Shoulder Taps:** While in the plank position, tap one hand to the opposite shoulder, alternating sides.

These essential body weight exercises, including push-ups, squats, and planks, form the foundation of a well-rounded workout routine. They are versatile, require no equipment, and can be adapted to your fitness level, making them suitable for beginners and experienced fitness enthusiasts alike. Incorporating these exercises into your routine will help you build strength, improve posture, and enhance your overall fitness.

3.4 Lunges

Lunges are excellent body weight exercises for strengthening the lower body, particularly the quadriceps, hamstrings, glutes, and calves. They also help improve balance and coordination.

How to Perform Lunges:

1. Begin by standing with your feet hip-width apart.

2. Take a step forward with one leg while keeping your upper body straight.

3. Lower your body by bending both knees until your front thigh is parallel to the ground, and your rear knee hovers just above the floor.

4. Push through your front heel to return to the starting position.

5. Repeat on the other leg.

- **Walking Lunges:** Perform lunges while walking forward, alternating between legs with each step.

- **Reverse Lunges:** Instead of stepping forward, take a step backward with each lunge.

- **Lateral Lunges:** Step to the side, bending one knee while keeping the other leg straight, and then return to the starting position.

3.5 Burpees

Burpees are a full-body, high-intensity body weight exercise that combines strength and cardiovascular conditioning. They are great for improving endurance and burning calories.

How to Perform Burpees:

1. Begin in a standing position.

2. Drop into a squat position with your hands on the ground.

3. Kick your feet back into a push-up position.

4. Perform a push-up (optional).

5. Quickly return your feet to the squat position.

6. Explode up from the squat, reaching your arms overhead.

7. Repeat the sequence as many times as desired.

Variations:

- **Modified Burpees:** To make burpees easier, you can omit the push-up or step back instead of jumping back.

- **Burpee Variations:** You can add variations like a tuck jump at the end of the movement or a 180-degree jump.

3.6 Dips

Dips are a fantastic body weight exercise for targeting the triceps, chest, and shoulders. They are particularly effective for building upper body strength and can be done using parallel bars, a bench, or even a sturdy chair.

How to Perform Dips:

1. Find parallel bars or a stable surface, such as the edges of two sturdy chairs, at shoulder-width distance.

2. Hold onto the bars or chair edges with your palms facing down.

3. Lower your body by bending your elbows until your shoulders are at or just below elbow level.

4. Push through your palms to
    straighten your arms and return to
    the starting position.

Variations:

- **Bench Dips:** These are a
  beginner-friendly variation where
  you perform dips using a bench or
  a low, stable surface.

- **Weighted Dips:** To increase the
  challenge, you can use a weight
  belt or hold a dumbbell between
  your knees.

- **Assisted Dips:** If you're working
  on building strength, you can use
  a resistance band or have a spotter
  assist you with the movement.

Incorporating lunges, burpees, and dips
into your body weight exercise routine
adds variety and targets different muscle
groups, providing a more comprehensive
workout. These exercises can help you
build strength, improve cardiovascular

fitness, and enhance overall functional fitness. As with any exercise, be sure to maintain proper form and adjust the intensity to match your fitness level.

3.7 Wall Sits

Wall sits are a simple yet effective isometric body weight exercise that primarily targets the quadriceps, hamstrings, and glutes. They are great for building leg strength and endurance while improving your ability to hold static positions.

How to Perform Wall Sits:

1. Find a clear wall or flat surface and stand with your back against it.

2. Slowly slide your body down the wall, bending your knees until they are at a 90-degree angle or slightly higher.

3. Keep your back flat against the wall and your thighs parallel to the ground.

4. Hold this position for as long as you can while keeping good form.

Variations:

- **One-Legged Wall Sits:** Lift one leg off the ground and hold the wall sit position on a single leg to increase the intensity.

- **Weighted Wall Sits:** Hold a weight (e.g., a dumbbell or a kettlebell) against your chest to add resistance.

3.8 Crunches

Crunches are a popular body weight exercise for strengthening the abdominal muscles, particularly the rectus abdominis (the "six-pack" muscles). They are effective for core stability and can help with posture and reducing the risk of lower back pain.

How to Perform Crunches:

1. Lie on your back with your knees bent and your feet flat on the floor.

2. Place your hands behind your head or cross your arms over your chest without pulling on your neck.

3. Contract your abdominal muscles to lift your upper body off the ground, bringing your shoulders toward your knees.

4. Keep your lower back on the ground and avoid pulling your head or neck with your hands.

5. Lower your upper body back to the ground with control.

Variations:

- **Reverse Crunches:** Instead of lifting your upper body, you lift your hips and lower back off the ground, engaging the lower abdominals.

- **Oblique Crunches:** Perform crunches with a twisting motion to target the oblique muscles. Bring your elbow toward the opposite knee.

- **Decline Crunches:** Elevate your feet on a bench or stable surface to increase the difficulty of the exercise.

Incorporating wall sits and crunches into your body weight exercise routine offers a well-rounded workout that addresses both lower body and core strength. These exercises can be performed with minimal space and no equipment, making them accessible for individuals looking to improve leg and abdominal strength and endurance. Ensure proper form and adjust the difficulty as needed to match your fitness level.

CHAPTER 4

Workout Routines

4.1 Beginner's Full-Body Routine

A beginner's full-body routine is a great starting point for those new to body weight exercises. This routine focuses on developing overall strength, flexibility, and endurance. It's essential to perform each exercise with proper form, and as you progress, you can gradually increase the number of repetitions and sets.

Warm-up:

- 5-10 minutes of light cardio (e.g., jumping jacks, jogging in place).

- Dynamic stretches to warm up your muscles (e.g., arm circles, leg swings).

Beginner's Full-Body Routine:

1. **Push-Ups** (3 sets of 8-10 reps): Start with knee push-ups if necessary and progress to standard push-ups as you gain strength.

2. **Squats** (3 sets of 10-12 reps): Focus on maintaining good form, and increase the depth as you become more comfortable.

3. **Planks** (3 sets of 20-30 seconds): Hold the plank position for as long as you can with proper form.

4. **Lunges** (3 sets of 10 reps per leg): Perform 10 lunges on one leg, then switch to the other leg.

5. **Wall Sits** (3 sets of 20-30 seconds): Hold the wall sit position for as long as you can while maintaining good form.

Cool-down:

- 5-10 minutes of static stretching for major muscle groups.

- Deep breathing exercises to help relax and cool down your body.

4.2 Core Strength Workout

A core strength workout is essential for building a strong and stable midsection. A strong core contributes to better posture, balance, and overall functional strength. This routine focuses on exercises that target the abdominal muscles and the lower back.

Warm-up:

- 5-10 minutes of light cardio.

- Dynamic stretches for the core, such as torso twists and hip circles.

Core Strength Workout:

1. **Crunches** (3 sets of 15-20 reps):
    Perform standard crunches or
    choose from variations like
    reverse crunches or oblique
    crunches.

2. **Planks** (3 sets of 30-60 seconds):
    Hold the plank position for
    progressively longer intervals as
    your core strength improves.

3. **Leg Raises** (3 sets of 10-12 reps):
    Lie on your back and raise your
    legs, keeping them straight, to
    work the lower abdominals.

4. **Superman** (3 sets of 10-12 reps):
    Lie face down, raise your arms,
    chest, and legs off the ground to
    engage the lower back and erector
    spinae muscles.

5. **Russian Twists** (3 sets of 10-12
    reps per side): Sit on the ground,
    lean back slightly, and rotate your
    torso to work the obliques.

Cool-down:

- 5-10 minutes of static stretching for the core and lower back.

- Deep breathing and relaxation exercises to promote recovery.

Progress gradually in terms of intensity, adding more sets, repetitions, or incorporating more challenging variations of exercises as your core strength improves. Maintaining proper form is crucial to avoid injury and maximize the benefits of your core strength workout.

4.3 Upper Body Strength Routine

An upper body strength routine focuses on developing the muscles in your chest, back, shoulders, and arms. This routine can help you build upper body strength, improve posture, and enhance your ability to perform everyday tasks.

Warm-up:

- 5-10 minutes of light cardio to raise your heart rate.

- Dynamic stretches for the upper body, such as arm circles and shoulder rolls.

Upper Body Strength Routine:

1. **Push-Ups** (3 sets of 8-10 reps): Perform standard or modified push-ups, gradually progressing to more challenging variations.

2. **Dips** (3 sets of 8-10 reps): Use parallel bars or a stable surface to target the triceps, chest, and shoulders.

3. **Pull-Ups or Inverted Rows** (3 sets of 8-10 reps): Use a pull-up bar or a sturdy horizontal bar to

target the back, biceps, and
shoulders.

4. **Bench Press** (3 sets of 8-10 reps):
If you have access to a bench,
perform bench presses to further
work the chest and shoulders.

5. **Planks** (3 sets of 30-60 seconds):
Strengthen the core and upper
body with plank variations.

Cool-down:

- 5-10 minutes of static stretching
for the upper body, focusing on
the chest, back, shoulders, and
arms.

- Deep breathing and relaxation
exercises to promote recovery.

4.4 Lower Body Strength Routine

A lower body strength routine concentrates on developing the muscles in your legs, including the quadriceps, hamstrings, glutes, and calves. Strengthening the lower body is essential for activities like walking, running, and maintaining overall mobility.

Warm-up:

- 5-10 minutes of light cardio to increase circulation.

- Dynamic leg stretches like leg swings and hip circles.

Lower Body Strength Routine:

1. **Squats** (3 sets of 10-12 reps): Perform body weight squats or add resistance as you progress.

2. **Lunges** (3 sets of 10 reps per leg):
   Step forward into lunges,
   alternating between legs.

3. **Calf Raises** (3 sets of 12-15 reps):
   Stand on your tiptoes and lower
   your heels to work the calf
   muscles.

4. **Wall Sits** (3 sets of 30-60
   seconds): Strengthen the
   quadriceps and glutes with this
   isometric exercise.

5. **Leg Press (if equipment
   available)** (3 sets of 8-10 reps): If
   you have access to a leg press
   machine, use it to target the entire
   lower body.

Cool-down:

- 5-10 minutes of static stretching
  for the legs, emphasizing the
  quadriceps, hamstrings, glutes,
  and calves.

- Deep breathing and relaxation exercises to facilitate recovery.

In both upper and lower body strength routines, focus on proper form and gradually increase the intensity as your strength and fitness level improve. These routines can be adjusted to suit your specific goals and preferences, and they can be performed with minimal equipment, making them accessible for a wide range of individuals.

CHAPTER 5

Progression and Modifications

5.1 Increasing Intensity

As you progress in your body weight exercise routine, it's important to continually challenge your muscles and fitness level by increasing the intensity of your workouts. Doing so not only keeps your workouts engaging but also helps you achieve your fitness goals more effectively. Here are some strategies to increase the intensity of your body weight exercises:

1. **Progressive Overload:** This fundamental principle of strength training involves gradually increasing the resistance or difficulty of your exercises. You

can achieve this by adding more repetitions, sets, or time to your exercises, or by increasing the complexity of the movements.

2. **Variations and Progressions:** Many body weight exercises have variations that make them more challenging. For example, you can progress from knee push-ups to standard push-ups or from regular squats to pistol squats. Explore these variations as you become more confident and capable.

3. **Time Under Tension:** Slow down the tempo of your exercises to increase time under tension. This can make body weight exercises significantly more challenging. For instance, perform push-ups and squats with a slow eccentric (lowering) phase and an explosive concentric (lifting) phase.

4. **Isometric Holds:** Incorporate isometric holds into your exercises. This involves pausing in a specific position of a movement, such as holding the bottom of a squat or pausing at the top of a push-up. Isometric holds engage your muscles for a longer duration, increasing the challenge.

5. **Decrease Rest Time:** Shorten the rest intervals between sets to keep your heart rate elevated and challenge your cardiovascular system. Reducing rest time forces your muscles to work harder to recover for the next set.

6. **Combine Exercises:** Create compound movements or superset exercises. For example, perform push-ups immediately followed by body weight squats, or lunges followed by planks. Combining exercises challenges different

muscle groups and increases overall intensity.

7. **Interval Training:** Incorporate high-intensity interval training (HIIT) into your routine. HIIT involves alternating between short bursts of intense exercise and brief recovery periods. This is an excellent way to boost cardiovascular fitness and overall intensity.

8. **Utilize Props:** If you have access to equipment like resistance bands, stability balls, or suspension trainers, you can integrate these tools into your body weight exercises to increase resistance and add variety to your workouts.

9. **Increase Range of Motion:** Work on improving your range of motion in various exercises. For example, in squats, aim to squat

deeper, or in push-ups, strive to touch your chest to the ground. This not only increases difficulty but also enhances joint mobility and flexibility.

10. **Frequency and Volume:** Gradually increase the frequency of your workouts and the total volume (number of sets and repetitions) over time. This progressive approach helps you adapt to higher training loads.

Increasing the intensity of your workouts should be done gradually to prevent overtraining and reduce the risk of injury. Listen to your body, stay consistent, and adjust your routines as needed to continue making progress in your fitness journey.

5.2 Incorporating Variations

Variations of body weight exercises can add diversity to your workout routine, challenge different muscle groups, and prevent exercise monotony. Here are some ways to incorporate variations into your workouts:

1. **Exercise Progressions:** Progress from simpler versions of exercises to more advanced ones. For example, if you're doing knee push-ups, work towards performing standard push-ups, and eventually, try one-arm push-ups.

2. **Exercise Regressions:** On the other hand, if you're finding an exercise too challenging, you can regress to a simpler version. For instance, if regular push-ups are too difficult, start with incline push-ups.

3. **Changing Hand or Foot Placement:** Alter the positioning of your hands or feet to emphasize different muscle groups. For example, placing your hands closer together during push-ups targets the triceps more, while a wider hand placement focuses on the chest.

4. **Varying Repetition Speed:** Adjust the tempo of your exercises. Slowing down the eccentric (lowering) phase of the movement increases time under tension and intensifies the exercise.

5. **Adding Isometric Holds:** Integrate pauses or isometric holds into your exercises. For instance, you can pause at the bottom of a squat or hold a halfway position during a pull-up.

6. **One-Leg or One-Arm Variations:** Incorporate exercises that challenge your balance and stability by using one limb at a time. Examples include one-legged squats (pistol squats) and one-arm push-ups.

7. **Combining Movements:** Create combinations of exercises to challenge multiple muscle groups simultaneously. For instance, combine push-ups with mountain climbers or squats with jump squats.

8. **Plyometric Variations:** Add explosive, jumping movements to your exercises. For example, perform explosive push-ups where you lift your hands off the ground at the top of the push-up or incorporate jump lunges.

9. **Directional Changes:** Instead of performing exercises in a linear

fashion, incorporate lateral
movements or diagonal motions
to engage different muscle fibers.

10. **Body Position Changes:** Explore
exercises that involve different
body positions, like planking on
your side, or exercises that
involve hanging from a pull-up
bar or rings.

11. **Grip Variations:** Change your
hand grip in exercises like pull-
ups. Using a neutral grip (palms
facing each other) or a wide grip
can target different parts of your
back and arms.

12. **Time-Based Variations:**
Implement timed intervals for
exercises, such as Tabata
intervals, where you perform an
exercise for 20 seconds with 10
seconds of rest.

13. **Elevated or Declined Variations:** Modify exercises by using an elevated or declined surface. For instance, decline push-ups or incline planks can challenge your body in different ways.

14. **Equipment and Props:** If you have access to equipment like resistance bands, stability balls, or parallettes, incorporate them into your body weight exercises to increase resistance and variability.

15. **Change the Surface:** Performing exercises on different surfaces like grass, sand, or an unstable platform can challenge your balance and engage more stabilizing muscles.

Incorporating variations into your body weight exercise routine not only keeps your workouts interesting but also helps prevent plateaus and stimulates muscle growth. Experiment with different variations to find what works best for your goals and preferences, and always prioritize proper form and safety.

5.3 Tracking Your Progress

Tracking your progress in your body weight exercise journey is crucial for several reasons. It helps you stay motivated, monitor your improvements, and make informed adjustments to your workout routine. Here's how to effectively track your progress:

1. **Keep a Workout Journal:** Maintain a dedicated workout journal or use a fitness app to record your workouts. Include details such as the exercises you performed, the number of sets and repetitions, and any modifications or variations you used. This written record can serve as a

valuable reference to track your progress.

2. **Set Clear Goals:** As mentioned earlier in the guide, setting clear and achievable goals is essential. Write down your fitness goals and make them specific, measurable, and time-bound. Regularly review and update your goals to reflect your evolving fitness aspirations.

3. **Take Before and After Photos:** Periodically take photos of yourself in the same poses and lighting conditions to visually assess changes in your physique over time. These photos can provide a tangible reminder of your progress.

4. **Measurements and Body Metrics:** Keep track of body measurements, such as waist circumference, hip circumference, and body weight. Monitor these

metrics at consistent intervals
(e.g., every two weeks or
monthly) to observe changes.

5. **Fitness Tests:** Incorporate fitness
   tests into your routine to gauge
   improvements in strength,
   endurance, and flexibility. For
   instance, track how many push-
   ups or pull-ups you can perform,
   measure your plank endurance, or
   test your flexibility using specific
   stretches.

6. **Use a Training Log:** Many
   fitness apps and websites offer
   training logs or templates for
   tracking workouts. These tools
   can help you record and visualize
   your progress more easily.

7. **Consistent Timing:** Schedule
   your workouts at the same time of
   day whenever possible. This can
   help ensure that you're comparing

your performance under similar conditions.

8. **Progression Data:** Pay attention to the progression of exercises. Note how you're advancing from easier variations to more challenging ones, whether you're increasing the number of sets and repetitions, or if you're performing exercises with better form.

9. **RPE (Rate of Perceived Exertion):** After each workout, rate your perceived level of exertion on a scale of 1 to 10. This subjective measure helps you gauge the intensity of your workouts and how they feel relative to your capabilities.

10. **Celebrate Achievements:** Acknowledge and celebrate your achievements, no matter how small they may seem. This

positive reinforcement can boost your motivation and commitment to your fitness journey.

11. **Adjustments and Adaptations:** Review your progress regularly and adjust your workouts accordingly. If you notice a plateau, consider changing exercises, intensifying your routines, or addressing areas that need improvement.

12. **Consult a Trainer or Coach:** Seeking the guidance of a fitness professional can provide valuable insights into your progress and help you make necessary adjustments to your routine.

Tracking your progress is a personalized process, and what works for one person may not be suitable for another. The key is to find a method that keeps you accountable, motivated, and engaged in your body weight exercise journey.

Regularly assessing your progress ensures that you're moving toward your fitness goals and making the most of your efforts.

CHAPTER 6

Nutritional Tips

6.1 Fueling Your Workouts

Proper nutrition is essential to fuel your body for effective workouts, whether you're engaging in body weight exercises or any other form of physical activity. Here are some tips for fueling your workouts:

1. **Pre-Workout Nutrition:**

   - Consume a balanced meal 1-2 hours before your workout. Include carbohydrates for energy, protein for muscle support, and a small amount of healthy fats.

- Opt for easily digestible foods to prevent discomfort during exercise.

- Snack on a banana or yogurt 30 minutes before a workout if you need quick energy.

2. **Stay Hydrated:**

- Dehydration can negatively impact your performance. Drink water throughout the day and before and during your workout.

- For longer workouts or intense sessions, consider sports drinks to replenish electrolytes lost through sweat.

3. **Post-Workout Nutrition:**

- Consume a combination of carbohydrates and protein within 1-2 hours after your workout to aid recovery and muscle repair.

- Options include a protein shake, a turkey sandwich, or a balanced meal with lean protein and complex carbohydrates.

4. **Timing Matters:**

- Tailor your nutrition to the time of day you work out. Morning exercisers may benefit from a light breakfast, while those working out in the evening can have a heartier meal.

5. **Personalized Approach:**

- Experiment with different foods and meal timing to find what works best for your body. Everyone's digestive system and preferences are unique.

6.2 Hydration

Proper hydration is fundamental for overall health and workout performance. Here's how to stay adequately hydrated:

1. **Monitor Water Intake:**

   - Pay attention to your daily water consumption. Aim for at least 8-10 glasses (64-80 ounces) of water per day, but individual needs may vary based on activity levels and climate.

2. **Pre-Workout Hydration:**

   - Drink 16-20 ounces of water 2-3 hours before your workout to ensure you're adequately hydrated.

3. **During Exercise:**

   - Sip water during your
     workout, especially if it's
     longer than 60 minutes.
     Listen to your body's
     signals for thirst and
     hydration needs.

4. **After Exercise:**

   - Rehydrate after your
     workout to replenish fluid
     losses. Water is usually
     sufficient unless you've
     engaged in a particularly
     long or intense session.

5. **Electrolytes:**

   - In hot or humid conditions
     or during extended
     exercise, consider
     beverages with added
     electrolytes or consume a
     small snack with

electrolyte-rich foods like
bananas or oranges.

6. **Limit Dehydrating Beverages:**

- Minimize the consumption
  of caffeinated and
  alcoholic beverages, as
  they can contribute to
  dehydration.

6.3 Balanced Diet for Fitness

A balanced diet is crucial for maintaining
overall health and supporting your
fitness goals. Here are some dietary tips
for staying on track:

1. **Macronutrient Balance:**

- Consume a mix of
  carbohydrates, proteins,
  and fats. Carbs provide
  energy, proteins support

muscle repair, and healthy fats are essential for overall health.

2. **Lean Protein:**

    - Prioritize lean sources of protein like chicken, turkey, fish, lean beef, tofu, and legumes. Protein is essential for muscle recovery and growth.

3. **Complex Carbohydrates:**

    - Include complex carbohydrates such as whole grains, fruits, vegetables, and legumes in your diet. These provide sustained energy for your workouts.

4. **Healthy Fats:**

    - Incorporate sources of healthy fats like avocados,

nuts, seeds, and olive oil.
These fats are important
for overall health and may
assist with energy and
recovery.

5. **Fruits and Vegetables:**

- Load up on a variety of
  colorful fruits and
  vegetables. They are rich
  in vitamins, minerals, and
  antioxidants that support
  overall health and
  recovery.

6. **Moderation:**

- Practice portion control
  and moderation to manage
  calorie intake and prevent
  overeating.

7. **Balanced Meals:**

- Ensure each meal contains
  a balance of

macronutrients to provide
energy, support recovery,
and regulate appetite.

8. **Nutrient Timing:**

- Tailor your nutrient intake
  to your activity levels.
  Consume more
  carbohydrates before
  workouts and focus on
  protein and fats after
  workouts.

9. **Hydration:**

- As discussed in the
  previous section, maintain
  proper hydration by
  drinking water throughout
  the day.

10. **Whole Foods:**

- Choose whole,
  unprocessed foods over

processed and highly
sugared or salted options.

11. Personalized Approach:

- Your dietary needs may
vary based on factors like
age, gender, activity level,
and specific fitness goals.
Consider consulting with a
registered dietitian for
personalized guidance.

There is no one-size-fits-all approach to
nutrition. Tailor your diet to your
individual needs and preferences, and
don't forget to enjoy your meals and
make healthy eating a sustainable part of
your lifestyle.

CHAPTER 7

Recovery and Injury Prevention

7.1 Importance of Rest

Rest is a critical component of any fitness routine, including body weight exercise programs. Here's why rest is important for recovery and injury prevention:

1. **Muscle Repair and Growth:** During workouts, especially resistance training exercises like body weight exercises, you create micro-tears in your muscle fibers. Rest allows your body to repair and rebuild these tissues, leading to muscle growth and increased strength.

2. **Energy Replenishment:** Exercise depletes your energy stores, particularly glycogen in your muscles and liver. Rest allows your body to replenish these energy stores, ensuring you have the necessary fuel for your next workout.

3. **Prevention of Overtraining:** Overtraining occurs when you don't provide your body with enough rest between workouts. Over time, this can lead to decreased performance, increased risk of injury, and fatigue. Adequate rest helps prevent overtraining.

4. **Injury Recovery:** If you have minor injuries or muscle soreness, rest gives your body time to heal. Pushing through pain or working out with an injury can worsen the condition and lead to more prolonged recovery times.

5. **Immune System Support:**
Regular, intense exercise can
temporarily suppress the immune
system. Rest days help your
immune system recover and
reduce the risk of illness.

6. **Mental Health:** Rest is crucial
for mental well-being. It reduces
stress, anxiety, and burnout,
promoting better mental health
and enhancing your overall
quality of life.

7. **Prevention of Overuse Injuries:**
Overuse injuries occur when you
perform the same movements
repeatedly without sufficient
recovery time. Rest days allow
your body to adapt and reduce the
risk of overuse injuries.

8. **Improved Performance:**
Adequate rest improves exercise
performance by ensuring you are
physically and mentally prepared

for each workout. You'll be more focused and able to give your best effort.

9. **Injury Prevention:** Fatigue from insufficient rest can lead to poor form and technique, increasing the risk of injuries. Proper rest helps maintain good form and reduce the likelihood of exercise-related injuries.

10. **Long-Term Sustainability:** Building rest into your fitness routine ensures that you can sustain your exercise program over the long term. Avoiding burnout and injury helps you maintain consistency.

Rest doesn't necessarily mean complete inactivity. Active recovery, such as light stretching, walking, or low-intensity activities like yoga, can be part of your rest days. Listen to your body, pay attention to signs of overtraining or fatigue, and prioritize rest as an essential part of your overall fitness plan.

7.2 Stretching and Flexibility

Stretching and flexibility exercises are vital components of recovery and injury prevention in body weight exercise programs. Here's why they are important and how to incorporate them into your routine:

Importance of Stretching and Flexibility:

1. **Improved Range of Motion:** Regular stretching helps improve the flexibility of your muscles and joints, which can lead to a wider range of motion in your exercises.

2. **Injury Prevention:** Flexible muscles and joints are less prone to strains and tears. Stretching

helps prevent injuries related to muscle tightness and imbalance.

3. **Reduced Muscle Soreness:** Stretching can alleviate muscle soreness by increasing blood flow and relieving tension in the muscles.

4. **Enhanced Posture:** Stretching exercises can help correct posture issues by loosening tight muscles that may be pulling your body out of alignment.

5. **Stress Relief:** Stretching and flexibility exercises are also excellent for relaxation and stress relief. They can calm the mind and reduce tension.

Incorporating Stretching and Flexibility Exercises:

1. **Warm-Up and Cool-Down:** Always include a dynamic warm-up before your workout and static

stretching during your cool-down. Dynamic warm-up exercises prepare your body for exercise, while static stretching at the end helps with muscle recovery.

2. **Focus on Major Muscle Groups:** Pay particular attention to stretching major muscle groups, such as hamstrings, quadriceps, calves, hip flexors, and shoulders. Stretching these areas can improve overall flexibility.

3. **Hold Stretches:** When performing static stretches, hold each stretch for 15-30 seconds. Avoid bouncing or forcing your body into positions. Breathe deeply and relax into the stretch.

4. **Include Yoga and Pilates:** Yoga and Pilates are excellent practices for improving flexibility and

balance. Consider incorporating them into your weekly routine.

5. **Foam Rolling:** Foam rolling or self-myofascial release with a foam roller can help release muscle knots and improve tissue quality.

6. **Use Resistance Bands:** Resistance bands can be used to assist in stretching and can be especially helpful for targeting specific muscle groups.

7. **Regularity:** Stretching should be a regular part of your fitness routine. Aim to stretch at least a few times a week or after each workout.

8. **Avoid Overstretching:** While it's important to stretch, avoid overstretching, which can lead to injuries. Stretch to a point of mild discomfort, not pain.

9. **Personalized Approach:** Your flexibility needs may vary based on your body, your fitness goals, and your physical limitations. Customize your stretching routine to suit your needs.

10. **Professional Guidance:** If you're unsure about how to stretch properly or have specific flexibility goals, consider consulting with a physical therapist or a certified yoga instructor for guidance.

Incorporating stretching and flexibility exercises into your routine can improve your performance, reduce the risk of injury, and contribute to overall physical well-being. Make flexibility training a consistent and essential part of your body weight exercise program.

7.3 Dealing with Common Injuries

Injuries can happen during any form of exercise, including body weight workouts. Knowing how to deal with common injuries is essential for your safety and well-being. Here are some guidelines for managing and preventing injuries:

1. Sprains and Strains:

- **Immediate Response:** Rest, ice, compression, and elevation (RICE) is the initial treatment for most sprains and strains. Immobilize the affected area and use ice to reduce swelling. Compression with an elastic bandage and elevation can help with pain and swelling.

- **Recovery:** Follow the RICE protocol, and allow the injury to heal completely. Gentle range-of-

motion exercises and stretches can
be helpful as the injury begins to
improve.

2. Muscle Soreness (Delayed Onset Muscle Soreness - DOMS):

- **Prevention:** Gradually increase
  the intensity and duration of your
  workouts to reduce the risk of
  DOMS. Warm up before
  exercising, stay hydrated, and
  include stretching in your routine.

- **Management:** If you experience
  muscle soreness, try gentle
  stretching, foam rolling, and over-
  the-counter pain relievers like
  ibuprofen. Rest and recover
  before resuming intense exercise.

3. Overuse Injuries:

- **Prevention:** Avoid overtraining
  by incorporating rest days into
  your routine. Ensure proper form

and technique in exercises to prevent overuse injuries.

- **Management:** If you suspect an overuse injury, reduce the intensity or frequency of the aggravating activity. Consult a healthcare professional for a proper diagnosis and rehabilitation plan.

4. Tendonitis:

- **Prevention:** Pay attention to your body's signals, such as pain, discomfort, or inflammation. Avoid pushing through pain, as it can lead to tendonitis. Use proper technique and ensure that your form is correct.

- **Management:** Rest the affected area, apply ice, and consider using over-the-counter anti-inflammatory medications. Physical therapy may be

beneficial for chronic or severe
cases.

5. Joint Injuries:

- **Prevention:** Maintain good form
  in exercises to prevent joint
  injuries. Gradually increase the
  intensity of your workouts and
  use proper technique.

- **Management:** If you suspect a
  joint injury, rest, ice, and
  compress the affected area.
  Elevating the joint may help
  reduce swelling. Seek
  professional medical advice for
  accurate diagnosis and treatment.

6. Stress Fractures:

- **Prevention:** Incorporate rest days
  into your routine and avoid
  excessive repetitive impact.
  Ensure proper footwear and
  technique in exercises.

- **Management:** Stress fractures typically require rest to allow for proper healing. Consult a healthcare professional for guidance on rehabilitation and a safe return to exercise.

7. Chronic Conditions:

- If you have pre-existing medical conditions or chronic injuries, consult with a healthcare professional and potentially a physical therapist before starting a new exercise program. They can help you develop a safe and effective fitness plan.

General Tips for Dealing with Injuries:

- Always listen to your body. If something doesn't feel right, stop the exercise and seek guidance if needed.

- Consult with a healthcare professional for an accurate diagnosis and personalized treatment plan.

- Focus on injury prevention through proper form, technique, and gradual progression in your workouts.

- Prioritize rest, recovery, and flexibility as essential components of injury prevention and management.

- Be patient with the healing process. Rushing back into exercise can lead to re-injury.

Safety and injury prevention are crucial for a successful and sustainable fitness journey. Consult with healthcare professionals for specific injury management and prevention advice, and consider their recommendations when

resuming your body weight exercise
program after an injury.

CHAPTER 8

Staying Motivated

8.1 Setting Realistic Expectations

Setting realistic expectations is essential for maintaining motivation in your body weight exercise journey. Unrealistic goals can lead to frustration and disappointment. Here's how to set achievable expectations:

1. **Define Specific Goals:** Clearly articulate your fitness goals, whether it's weight loss, muscle gain, improved flexibility, or increased endurance. Specific goals give you a clear direction.

2. **Break Down Your Goals:** Divide your larger goals into smaller, manageable milestones.

Achieving these milestones can provide a sense of accomplishment and motivation.

3. **Consider Your Current Fitness Level:** Be realistic about where you currently stand in terms of fitness. Setting goals that are too ambitious for your current abilities can lead to frustration.

4. **Be Patient:** Understand that progress takes time. Rome wasn't built in a day, and neither is your fitness. Be patient with yourself and recognize that results may not be immediate.

5. **Track Your Progress:** Use a journal, fitness app, or regular assessments to monitor your progress. Celebrate your successes, even if they're small, and use setbacks as learning opportunities.

6. **Adjust as Needed:** It's okay to modify your goals as you progress and discover new interests or challenges. Adaptability can keep your motivation high.

7. **Consult a Professional:** If you're unsure about setting realistic goals, consider seeking guidance from a certified fitness trainer or a registered dietitian. They can help you align your expectations with your abilities and resources.

8.2 Creating a Routine

Establishing a routine is a key to staying motivated in your body weight exercise program. Routines provide structure and help make exercise a regular part of your life. Here's how to create an effective routine:

1. **Set a Schedule:** Choose specific days and times for your workouts

that align with your daily
schedule. Consistency is key.

2. **Plan Your Workouts:** Decide in
advance which exercises you'll do
during each workout. This
eliminates the need to figure it out
on the spot and helps you stay
focused.

3. **Include Rest Days:** Ensure your
routine includes rest days to allow
for recovery and prevent burnout
or overtraining.

4. **Gradual Progression:** Gradually
increase the intensity and
complexity of your workouts over
time. This keeps your routine
challenging and prevents plateaus.

5. **Variety:** Introduce variety into
your routine by changing
exercises, incorporating different
forms of exercise, or exploring
new challenges. This prevents

boredom and keeps things interesting.

6. **Warm-Up and Cool-Down:** Include warm-up and cool-down exercises in every workout to prepare your body for exercise and aid in recovery.

7. **Time Management:** Efficiently manage your workout time to make the most of your sessions. Avoid long breaks and stay focused during your routine.

8. **Incorporate Other Activities:** Don't limit your routine to exercise only. Incorporate activities like meditation, mindfulness, or goal-setting to boost motivation and overall well-being.

9. **Hold Yourself Accountable:** Share your routine with a workout buddy or post it publicly to hold

yourself accountable. Knowing someone is expecting you to exercise can be motivating.

8.3 Finding Accountability

Accountability is a powerful motivator in your fitness journey. It helps you stay on track and remain consistent. Here are ways to find accountability:

1. **Workout Buddy:** Partner with a friend or family member who shares your fitness goals. You can exercise together, support each other, and hold one another accountable.

2. **Join a Group Class:** Participating in group fitness classes can provide a sense of community and accountability. You're more likely to attend scheduled classes and stay committed.

3. **Personal Trainer:** Consider hiring a personal trainer for one-on-one guidance, support, and accountability. They can tailor workouts to your needs and keep you motivated.

4. **Fitness Apps and Online Communities:** Many fitness apps and online platforms offer virtual communities where you can track your progress, share your goals, and receive encouragement from like-minded individuals.

5. **Set Public Goals:** Announce your fitness goals to friends and family, either in person or on social media. Knowing that others are aware of your goals can boost your commitment.

6. **Accountability Partners:** Connect with an accountability partner, whether it's a friend, family member, or an online

accountability group. Share your progress, celebrate achievements, and provide support during challenging times.

7. **Track Your Progress:** Regularly assess and track your progress, whether through measurements, photos, or fitness assessments. Seeing your improvement can motivate you to keep going.

8. **Incentives and Rewards:** Create a reward system for achieving your fitness goals. Treat yourself to something enjoyable when you reach milestones, which can serve as a motivating factor.

Motivation can ebb and flow, so having multiple layers of accountability can help you stay on course during challenging periods. Find the combination of accountability methods that works best for you and keeps you motivated to pursue your fitness goals.